HOW TO STOP SNORING

A Comprehensive Guide to End Your Noisy Nights

By

Gail D. Jacob's

Introduction:

Are you tired of being woken up in the middle of the night by the sound of your own snoring? Do you feel exhausted in the morning, despite getting what should have been a full night's sleep? If so, you're not alone. Millions of people around the world suffer from snoring, a common sleep disorder that can have a significant impact on your quality of life.

Snoring occurs when the muscles in your throat relax too much during sleep, causing the airway to narrow and vibrate as air passes through. This can result in a loud, disruptive noise that can disturb your own sleep as well as that of your partner or other family members.

But snoring is not just an inconvenience; it can also have serious health consequences. Chronic snoring has been linked to a range of health issues, including high blood pressure, heart disease, and stroke. It can also disrupt the sleep of those around you, leading to irritability, mood swings, and relationship problems.

The good news is that there are many ways to stop snoring and get a good night's sleep. From simple lifestyle changes to medical interventions, there are a variety of approaches you can take to reduce or eliminate your snoring.

In this book, we'll explore the different causes of snoring and provide practical solutions to help you stop snoring and improve your sleep quality. We'll discuss lifestyle changes you can make, such as adjusting your sleeping position and managing nasal congestion, as well as review various anti-snoring devices and products that are available. We'll also cover medical interventions for snoring, such as surgery and CPAP therapy, and explain when these options might be necessary.

By the end of this book, you'll have a comprehensive understanding of snoring and the tools you need to address it. It's time to take control of your sleep and start waking up feeling rested and refreshed. Let's get started.

Contents;

- Discussion of how diet and exercise can affect snoring

- Tips for maintaining a healthy weight to reduce snoring

- Advice on avoiding alcohol and smoking to reduce snoring

Chapter 3: Sleeping Position

- Explanation of how sleeping position affects snoring

- Tips for adjusting sleeping position to reduce snoring

- Review of different types of anti-snoring pillows and devices that can help improve sleep position

Chapter 4: Nasal Congestion and Allergies

- Explanation of how nasal congestion and allergies can cause snoring

- Advice on how to manage nasal congestion and allergies to reduce snoring

- Review of different types of nasal sprays and allergy medication that can help alleviate snoring

Chapter 5: Devices and Products for Snoring Relief

- Overview of different types of anti-snoring devices and products,

including chin straps, nasal dilators, and mouthguards
- Explanation of how these products work to reduce snoring
- Review of the effectiveness and safety of different products

Chapter 6: Medical Interventions for Snoring
- Explanation of medical treatments for snoring, including surgery and Continuous Positive Airway Pressure (CPAP) therapy
- Discussion of the benefits and risks associated with these interventions

- Overview of the process for seeking medical treatment for snoring

- Encouragement for readers to take action to reduce their snoring and improve their sleep quality and overall health.

Chapter 1

Understanding Snoring

If you or a loved one suffers from snoring, it's important to understand what causes it in order to find an effective solution. In this chapter, we'll dive into the anatomy of the throat and explore the common causes of snoring.

Anatomy of the Throat

The throat is made up of various structures, including the soft palate, uvula, tonsils, and tongue. During sleep, the muscles in the throat naturally relax, which can cause these structures to narrow and vibrate as air passes through. This vibration is what creates the sound of snoring.

Types of Snoring

Not all snoring is the same. There are three main types of snoring: nasal snoring, mouth snoring, and tongue snoring.

Nasal snoring is caused by congestion in the nasal passages. This can be the result of allergies, a deviated septum, or other nasal issues.

Mouth snoring occurs when the muscles in the mouth and throat relax, causing the tongue to fall back and block the airway.

Tongue snoring is caused by the tongue obstructing the airway due to poor muscle tone or excess tissue.

Common Causes of Snoring

There are many factors that can contribute to snoring. Some of the most common causes include:

- Obesity: carrying excess weight can put pressure on the airway, leading to snoring.

- Aging: as we get older, the muscles in the throat naturally lose tone, making snoring more likely.

- Alcohol and sedatives: these substances can relax the muscles in the throat, leading to snoring.

- Sleep apnea: a sleep disorder characterized by pauses in breathing during sleep. Snoring is a common symptom of sleep apnea.

Snoring is a complex issue with many potential causes. By understanding the anatomy of the throat and the common factors that contribute to snoring, you can begin to explore effective solutions for addressing this problem. In the following chapters, we'll discuss lifestyle changes, anti-snoring devices, and medical interventions that can help you stop snoring and get the quality sleep you need.

Chapter 2

Lifestyle Changes to Reduce Snoring

If you're a chronic snorer, making some simple lifestyle changes may be enough to significantly reduce or even eliminate your snoring. In this chapter, we'll explore some of the most effective lifestyle changes you can make to reduce snoring.

Weight Loss

Carrying excess weight is one of the most common causes of snoring. Losing weight can help reduce the amount of pressure on the airway, making it easier to breathe during sleep. Even a small amount of weight loss can make a significant difference in reducing snoring.

Exercise

Regular exercise can help strengthen the muscles in the throat and improve overall respiratory function, reducing the likelihood of snoring. Aim for at least 30 minutes of moderate exercise per day, such as brisk walking, cycling, or swimming.

Sleep Position

Sleeping on your back can make snoring worse, as it allows the tongue and soft palate to fall back and obstruct the airway. Try sleeping on your side instead. You can also use a body pillow to keep yourself in the right position throughout the night.

Avoid Alcohol and Sedatives

Alcohol and sedatives can relax the muscles in the throat, leading to increased snoring. Avoid consuming these substances before bed, or limit your intake to earlier in the evening.

Manage Allergies and Congestion

Nasal congestion can lead to snoring, so it's important to manage any allergies or congestion you may have. Consider using a saline nasal spray, a humidifier, or taking an antihistamine to reduce congestion and improve breathing.

By making these simple lifestyle changes, you may be able to significantly reduce or even eliminate your snoring. In addition to these strategies, there are a number of anti-snoring devices and medical interventions that can also be effective

in addressing snoring. In the following
chapters, we'll explore these options in
more detail.

Chapter 3

Anti-Snoring Devices

If lifestyle changes alone aren't enough to reduce your snoring, you may want to consider using an anti-snoring device. There are many different types of devices on the market, each designed to address specific causes of snoring. In this chapter, we'll explore some of the most common anti-snoring devices and how they work.

Nasal Strips

Nasal strips are adhesive strips that you place on the outside of your nose. They work by gently pulling open the nasal passages, allowing for better airflow and reducing congestion. Nasal strips can be particularly effective for those with nasal snoring.

Mouthpieces

Mouthpieces, also known as mandibular advancement devices (MADs), work by holding the lower jaw and tongue forward, which helps to keep the airway open and reduce snoring. MADs are typically custom-fitted by a dentist or orthodontist, but there are also over-the-counter options available.

Tongue Retaining Devices

Tongue retaining devices (TRDs) work by holding the tongue in place to prevent it from falling back and obstructing the airway. TRDs are typically made of soft plastic and are custom-fitted by a dentist or orthodontist.

Positional Therapy Devices

Positional therapy devices are designed to help you maintain a specific sleep position throughout the night. These devices can include pillows, wedges, and even specialized shirts that are designed to prevent you from rolling onto your back.

CPAP Machines

Continuous positive airway pressure (CPAP) machines are medical devices that deliver a continuous stream of air through a mask, keeping the airway open and preventing snoring. CPAP machines are typically prescribed by a doctor for those with sleep apnea.

There are many different anti-snoring devices available, each designed to address specific causes of snoring. While these devices can be effective for many people, it's important to choose the right device for your needs and to use it properly in order to achieve the best results. In the following chapter, we'll explore medical interventions that can also be effective in treating snoring.

Chapter 4

Medical Interventions for Snoring

For some people, lifestyle changes and anti-snoring devices may not be enough to reduce snoring. In these cases, medical interventions may be necessary. In this chapter, we'll explore some of the most common medical interventions for snoring.

Palatal Implants

Palatal implants are small rods that are inserted into the soft palate to stiffen the tissue and reduce snoring.

This is a minor surgical procedure that is typically performed under local anesthesia in a doctor's office.

Radiofrequency Ablation

Radiofrequency ablation (RFA) is a minimally invasive procedure that uses heat to reduce the size of the tissues in the throat, reducing snoring. RFA is typically performed under local anesthesia and requires little recovery time.

Uvulopalatopharyngoplasty (UPPP)
UPPP is a surgical procedure that involves removing excess tissue from

the throat, including the uvula and soft palate. This procedure is typically performed under general anesthesia in a hospital setting and may require several weeks of recovery time.

Laser-Assisted Uvulopalatoplasty (LAUP)

LAUP is a laser-assisted procedure that is used to remove excess tissue from the throat. This is typically performed under local anesthesia in a doctor's office and requires minimal recovery time.

Maxillo-Mandibular Advancement (MMA) Surgery

MMA surgery involves moving the upper and lower jaws forward to create more space in the airway, reducing snoring. This is a major surgical procedure that is typically performed under general anesthesia in a hospital setting and requires several weeks of recovery time.

Medical interventions can be effective in reducing snoring, but they are typically reserved for those with severe snoring or sleep apnea. If you're considering a medical intervention for snoring, it's important to discuss the risks and benefits with your doctor to determine if it's the right option for you. In the next chapter, we'll explore some natural remedies and alternative therapies that can also be effective in reducing snoring.

Chapter 5

Natural Remedies and Alternative Therapies for Snoring

While lifestyle changes, anti-snoring devices, and medical interventions can be effective in reducing snoring, some people prefer to explore natural remedies and alternative therapies. In this chapter, we'll explore some of the most popular natural remedies and alternative therapies for snoring.

Essential Oils

Certain essential oils, such as eucalyptus, peppermint, and lavender, can help to open up the airways and reduce congestion, making it easier to breathe and reducing snoring. Essential oils can be diffused in a room, applied topically, or used in a steam inhalation.

Acupuncture

Acupuncture involves the insertion of small needles into specific points on the body to promote relaxation and reduce tension. This can help to reduce snoring by relaxing the muscles in the throat and improving airflow.

Yoga

Certain yoga poses, such as the lion pose and the fish pose, can help to strengthen the muscles in the throat and reduce snoring. Additionally, practicing yoga can help to promote relaxation and reduce stress, which can also contribute to better sleep and less snoring.

Honey

Honey has natural anti-inflammatory properties and can help to reduce inflammation in the throat, making it easier to breathe and reducing snoring. Simply add a spoonful of honey to a cup of warm water or tea before bed.

Weight Loss

Excess weight can contribute to snoring by putting pressure on the airways and obstructing breathing. Losing weight through a healthy diet and exercise can help to reduce snoring and improve overall health.

Natural remedies and alternative therapies can be effective in reducing snoring, particularly for those with mild to moderate snoring. However, it's important to note that not all natural remedies and alternative therapies are scientifically proven and some may not work for everyone. It's always a good idea to discuss any natural remedies or alternative therapies with your doctor before trying them. In the final chapter, we'll summarize the key takeaways from the book and provide some additional tips for reducing snoring.

Chapter 6

Tips and Tricks for Reducing Snoring

In this final chapter, we'll summarize the key takeaways from the book and provide some additional tips and tricks for reducing snoring.

1. Sleep on your side: Sleeping on your back can cause the tongue and soft palate to collapse to the back of the throat, obstructing breathing and causing snoring. Sleeping on your side

can help to keep the airways open and reduce snoring.

2. Elevate your head: Elevating your head with a pillow or adjustable bed can help to reduce snoring by opening up the airways and reducing pressure on the throat.

3. Avoid alcohol and sedatives: Alcohol and sedatives can relax the muscles in the throat, increasing the likelihood of snoring. Avoiding these substances before bed can help to reduce snoring.

4. Stay hydrated: Dehydration can cause mucus to thicken and build up in the throat, contributing to snoring. Drinking plenty of water throughout the day can help to keep the throat hydrated and reduce snoring.

5. Practice good sleep hygiene: Practicing good sleep hygiene, such as sticking to a regular sleep schedule, creating a relaxing bedtime routine, and keeping your sleep environment cool, quiet, and dark, can help to improve sleep quality and reduce snoring.

6. Consider seeing a sleep specialist: If you have severe snoring or suspect that you may have sleep apnea, consider seeing a sleep specialist for further evaluation and treatment.

Snoring can be a frustrating and disruptive issue, but there are many lifestyle changes, anti-snoring devices, medical interventions, natural remedies, and alternative therapies that can help to reduce snoring. By making simple changes to your sleep habits and lifestyle, you can improve your sleep quality and reduce snoring, leading to better health and overall well-being.

Chapter 7

Lifestyle Changes for Better Sleep

Sleep is a vital part of a healthy lifestyle, yet it's often overlooked in our busy lives. While snoring prevention is important, there are many other lifestyle changes you can make to improve your sleep quality and overall health. In this chapter, we'll explore some tips for better sleep and how lifestyle changes can help you achieve it.

Tips for Improving Sleep Quality Beyond Snoring Prevention

1. Stick to a consistent sleep schedule: Go to bed and wake up at the same time every day, even on weekends. This helps regulate your body's sleep-wake cycle.

2. Create a relaxing bedtime routine: A calming routine before bed can signal to your body that it's time to wind down. This could include reading a book, taking a warm bath, or practicing relaxation techniques like deep breathing.

3. Make your bedroom a sleep haven: Keep your bedroom cool, dark, and quiet. Invest in comfortable bedding and pillows, and remove any distractions like electronics.

4. Limit caffeine and alcohol intake: Both caffeine and alcohol can disrupt sleep, so it's best to avoid them or consume them in moderation.

5. Get regular exercise: Regular physical activity can help you fall asleep faster and enjoy deeper sleep.

Just make sure to avoid exercising too close to bedtime.

How Lifestyle Changes Can Improve Sleep Quality and Overall Health

Poor sleep quality can have a significant impact on your health, leading to a range of issues including fatigue, irritability, and poor concentration. Making positive lifestyle changes can improve your sleep quality and have a positive impact on your overall health. Here are a few ways that lifestyle changes can help:

1. Reduced stress: Chronic stress can make it difficult to fall asleep and stay asleep. Engaging in relaxation techniques like meditation or yoga can help reduce stress levels and promote better sleep.

2. Improved diet: Eating a balanced diet can help regulate your sleep-wake cycle and provide your body with the nutrients it needs to support healthy sleep.

3. Enhanced physical health: Regular exercise and healthy lifestyle habits like not smoking and limiting alcohol intake can help reduce the risk of conditions like obesity, heart disease, and diabetes that can negatively affect sleep.

Review of the Importance of Good Sleep Hygiene

Good sleep hygiene refers to the habits and practices that promote good sleep. These habits can include sticking to a consistent sleep schedule, creating a relaxing sleep environment, and avoiding stimulating activities before bed. Good sleep hygiene is important for maintaining healthy sleep patterns and improving overall health. Poor sleep hygiene can lead to chronic sleep problems and negatively impact your physical and mental health.

Making lifestyle changes to improve your sleep quality can have a significant impact on your overall health and well-being. By implementing good sleep hygiene habits and making positive lifestyle changes, you can enjoy better sleep and all the benefits that come with it.

Conclusion

Snoring is a common issue that affects millions of people around the world. While it may seem like a minor annoyance, snoring can have a significant impact on sleep quality, daytime functioning, and overall health and well-being.

In this book, we've explored a range of strategies and techniques for reducing snoring, including lifestyle changes, anti-snoring devices, medical interventions, natural remedies, and alternative therapies. By understanding the underlying causes of snoring and implementing the right strategies for your individual needs, you can improve your sleep quality, reduce snoring, and enhance your overall health and well-being.

Remember that everyone's journey to better sleep is unique, and it may take some trial and error to find the strategies and techniques that work best for you. Be patient with yourself, and don't hesitate to seek professional help if you're struggling with severe snoring or other sleep issues.

We hope that this book has been helpful in providing you with the information and tools you need to reduce your snoring and improve your sleep quality. Here's to a good night's sleep!